FOOD FOR HEALTHY CONCEPTION
How Nutrition Can Impact Your Fertility Journey

GLEN ROBERT

Table of content

Chapter 1.

Why you should have real food for healthy conception

Consuming a healthy, well-balanced, nutrient-rich diet is crucial for the health of moms-to-be and their babies. While pregnancy nutrition isn't a one-size-fits-all approach, there are some key concepts to keep in mind when eating during pregnancy.

Defining Real Food
In general, eating "real food" is considered a healthy practice. However, the definition of real food is a gray area within nutrition. Here are a few ways to evaluate how "real" your diet is.

- Nutrient-rich foods, also referred to as nutrient-dense foods, contain many nutrients. Nutrients are broken down into two categories: Macronutrients, which include carbohydrates, proteins, and fats, and micronutrients, which include vitamins and minerals.If a food is high in vitamins, minerals, fiber, protein, and/or healthy fatty acids, it is considered nutrient-rich. On the flip side, if the food does not contain many of these components, it is considered nutrient-poor. Most real foods are nutrient-dense foods that help nourish your body.

- Whole foods are foods that are consumed in a similar form to how they appear in nature. Most whole foods do not contain added sugars, processed carbohydrates, added colors or flavors, or other manufactured ingredients. Most whole foods are naturally nutrient-dense; real foods include fruits, vegetables, nuts, seeds, beans, dairy, meat, poultry, and seafood.

- Unprocessed foods, like whole foods, are not modified and they appear similar to how they do in nature. In our society, many foods are processed until they are barely recognizable from their original form, and wouldn't fit the real food definition.

Why Real Foods during Pregnancy?

Consuming real, nutrient-dense, whole foods gives your body the nourishment it needs to grow a healthy baby. As a mom with healthy food intake and healthy nutrient stores, your baby's health will be optimized as well. Real foods also help protect against anemia during pregnancy and reduce the risk of pregnancy complications including gestational diabetes, preeclampsia (high blood pressure), and preterm labor. Optimizing your diet during pregnancy also helps with postpartum recovery.

A Well-Balanced Pregnancy Diet

You can use these concepts to build a healthy, well-balanced pregnancy diet. Well-balanced meals and snacks are an important part of a healthy diet for everyone, but even more important during pregnancy. Generally, combining real foods into nourishing meals and snacks is a healthy way to approach nourishing your body throughout pregnancy.

In general, eat a varied diet that contains nutrient-dense foods including:

- Fruits and vegetables for micronutrients and fiber.
- Complex carbohydrates for iron, B vitamins, folate, and fiber.
- Lean proteins to support your baby's optimal growth and development.

- Healthy fats to meet your energy needs and support your baby's brain development.

Certain micronutrients are even more important during pregnancy. Some essential nutrients include:

- Vitamin A for your baby's eyes and immune system.
- Vitamin D for your baby's bone development.
- Calcium to work with vitamin D to form your baby's teeth, bones, muscles, heart, and nerves.
- Choline for your baby's brain development.
- Folate for your baby's developing brain and spinal cord.
- Iron to support your increased blood supply as a mom-to-be.

Simple Changes

While it is helpful to know what you should eat, it's also helpful to know what foods to limit. Generally, limiting processed foods is best for everyone, but especially for pregnant women hoping to optimize their diets. Instead of trying to avoid whole food groups, make small changes within each food group to make your diet more real food-based.

- Fruits and vegetables consumed in their whole form are the most nutrient-dense. Frozen fruits and vegetables also retain their nutrients, and are a great option. Unsweetened dried fruit also provides beneficial nutrients. However, be sure to look for unsweetened and no-added -sugar options to avoid added sugars. Fruit snacks, veggie chips, and other processed foods that seem to contain fruits and vegetables, but really don't, should be limited.

- Carbohydrates fall into two main categories – whole grains and refined grains. Whole grains include whole-wheat bread and pasta, brown rice, oats, and quinoa. These grains are less processed and contain more beneficial nutrients. Refined grains are white bread, pasta, and rice, which are much more processed and lower in nutrients. Try choosing whole grains as often as possible.

- Proteins that are minimally processed are generally considered the healthiest protein options. Limiting processed meats (bacon, sausage) helps improve your overall diet quality.Lean cuts of beef or pork, poultry, and seafood are all good sources of protein during pregnancy. Plant-based proteins such as tofu and beans are also healthy choices.

- Eggs and dairy products are also beneficial healthy, whole foods during pregnancy. Consuming whole eggs and whole-milk dairy also helps improve overall nutrient intake. Eggs are one of the only dense food sources of choline, which is crucial for your baby's brain. Eating the whole egg provides you with the most choline. Consuming full-fat, whole-milk dairy provides your body with the fat needed to absorb vitamins A, D, E, and K.

- Healthy fats are an important contributor to your overall energy needs during pregnancy. Specifically, omega-3 fatty acids are necessary for healthy fetal brain development. Even more specifically, the omega-3 fatty acid docosahexaenoic acid (DHA) is crucial for your baby's brain formation. Nuts, seeds, avocado, and fatty fish are all great sources of healthy fats during pregnancy. Although fish and shellfish are good sources of protein, healthy fats, and iron, there are risks of consuming certain types of seafood that may be high in mercury while pregnant.

Staying Realistic

While sticking to these recommendations would be ideal, pregnancy may pose challenges to getting the nutrients your body needs. Food cravings are common and may influence your food choices throughout your pregnancy. Food aversions are also common and may make some of the foods you know are healthy unrealistic for you at certain points in your pregnancy.

While it's not a food, your prenatal vitamin is a key part of ensuring you are getting the nutrients you need regardless of what foods are realistic for you day-to-day. Prenatal vitamins provide you and your baby with the nutrients that are essential for pregnancy to ensure you are getting them daily. However, the nutrients in your food have a synergistic effect, and getting your nutrients from foods is generally preferred to consuming them in food supplements. Continue taking your prenatal, but do your best to eat a variety of real foods too. If you need support in deciding which prenatal to take, talk to your doctor or dietitian.

Chapter 2.

Nutrients for healthy conception

Becoming healthy before becoming pregnant

Preconception nutrition is a vital part of preparing for pregnancy. Factors such as your weight compared with your height and what you eat can play an important role in your health during pregnancy and the health of your developing fetus.

Pre-pregnancy weight

Your pre-pregnancy weight directly influences your baby's birth weight. Studies show that underweight women are more likely to give birth to small babies, even though they may gain the same amount in pregnancy as normal weight women. Overweight women have increased risks for problems in pregnancy such as gestational diabetes or high blood pressure. Talk with your healthcare provider about whether you need to lose or gain weight before becoming pregnant.

Pre-pregnancy nutrition

Many women don't eat a well-balanced diet before pregnancy and may not have the proper nutritional status for the demands of pregnancy. Generally, a pregnant woman needs to add about 300 extra calories daily after the first trimester to meet the needs of her body and her developing fetus. But those calories, as well as her entire diet, need to be healthy, balanced, and nutritious.

The MyPlate icon is a guideline to help you eat a healthy diet by encouraging a variety of foods while getting the right number of calories and fat. The USDA and the U.S.

Department of Health and Human Services have prepared this food plate to help you select a variety of healthy foods. MyPlate is available for pregnant and breastfeeding women.

The MyPlate icon is divided into 5 food group categories:

- Grains. Foods that are made from wheat, rice, oats, cornmeal, barley, or another cereal grain are grain products. Make at least half of your grains whole-grains. Examples of whole-grains include whole-wheat, brown rice, and oatmeal.
- Vegetables. Vary your vegetables. Choose a variety of vegetables, including dark green, red, and orange vegetables, legumes (dry beans and peas), and starchy vegetables. Healthier options include buying fresh, canned (low-sodium or no-salt-added versions) or plain

frozen (without added sauces or seasonings) vegetables.

- Fruits. Any fruit or 100% fruit juice counts as part of the fruit group. Fruits may be fresh, canned (packed in 100% juice or water), frozen, or dried, and may be whole, cut-up, or pureed.
- Dairy. Milk products and many foods made from milk are considered part of this food group. Use fat-free or low-fat dairy products that are high in calcium.
- Protein. Go lean with protein. Choose low-fat or lean meats and poultry. Vary your protein routine by choosing more fish, nuts, seeds, peas, and beans.
- Oils are not a food group, yet some, such as nut oils, contain key nutrients and should be included in the diet in moderation. Others, such as animal fats, are solid at room temperature and should be avoided.

Exercise and everyday physical activity should also be included with a healthy dietary plan.

In addition to the MyPlate food groups, include the following nutrients in your preconception diet and continued into pregnancy:

Folic acid

All women of childbearing age need 400 micrograms (0.4 mg) of folic acid each day. Folic acid is a nutrient found in some green leafy vegetables, nuts, beans, citrus fruits, fortified breakfast cereals, and some vitamin supplements. It can help reduce the risk of birth defects of the brain and spinal cord (called neural tube defects). The most common neural tube defect is spina bifida, in which the vertebrae don't fuse together properly, causing the spinal cord to be exposed. This can lead to varying degrees of paralysis, incontinence, and, sometimes, intellectual disability.

Folic acid is most beneficial during the first 28 days after conception, when most neural tube defects occur. Unfortunately, many women don't realize they are pregnant until 28 days. This is why it's important to start folic acid before conception and continue through pregnancy. Your healthcare provider will recommend the right amount of folic acid to meet your needs.

Most healthcare providers will prescribe a prenatal supplement before conception, or shortly afterward, to ensure all of your nutritional needs are met. However, a prenatal supplement does not replace a healthy diet.

Iron

Many women have low iron stores as a result of monthly menstruation and diets low in iron. Building iron stores helps prepare a mother's body for the needs of the fetus during pregnancy. Good sources of iron include the following:

Meats such as beef, pork, lamb, liver, and other organ meats.
Poultry such as chicken, duck, and turkey (especially dark meat).
Fish and shellfish including sardines, anchovies, clams, mussels, and oysters. Check with your healthcare provider before consuming other types of fish as some may contain high levels of mercury.
Leafy greens of the cabbage family such as broccoli, kale, turnip greens, and collards.
Legumes such as lima beans and green peas, dry beans and peas such as pinto beans and black-eyed peas, and canned baked beans.
Whole-grain breads and iron-enriched white bread, pasta, rice, and cereals.

Calcium

Preparing for pregnancy includes building healthy bones. If there is not enough calcium in the pregnancy diet, the fetus may draw calcium from the mother's bones, which can put women at risk for osteoporosis later in life. The recommended calcium intake for women is 1,000 milligrams. Three servings of milk or other dairy products each day equals about 1,000 milligrams of calcium.

Always talk with your healthcare provider about your healthy diet and exercise needs.

Chapter 3.

Foods for healthy pregnancy

You may have heard that your eating habits may change during pregnancy. That's OK! You will find foods that you like and that are healthy for both you and your baby. Eating nutritious foods will help you support your pregnancy and the new changes in your body.

Healthy eating during pregnancy includes knowing how much to eat and what foods are healthy. It's also finding a balance between getting enough nutrients for your baby's growth and keeping a healthy weight for you and your baby's health. Nutrients are the building blocks of the body like protein, carbohydrates and fat. Talk to your provider about how you can get the nutrients you need in your diet.

What nutrients do I need during pregnancy to keep my baby and me healthy?

During pregnancy, you can get a lot of nutrients from different sources or food groups such as grains, proteins, vegetables, fruits, and dairy. Other sources of nutrients are fats and vitamins and minerals.

Proteins help your body with muscle and tissue growth and also with your baby's growth. Protein can be found in foods like:

- Beef, pork, fish and poultry
- Eggs
- Milk, cheese and other dairy foods
- Beans and peas
- Nuts and Seeds

- Soy products like tempeh and tofu

Carbohydrates are found in food like grains and they're your body's fuel to help you do your activities. There are different types of carbohydrates. Foods can have a combination of all three types of carbohydrates.

Simple carbohydrates are broken down fast, spiking your blood sugar quickly. It's best to limit foods high in simple carbohydrates like:

- Table sugar
- Certain breakfast cereals
- Sugary desserts

Complex carbohydrates give longer lasting energy and can be found in:

- Whole grain products, like bread, rice and pasta
- Beans
- Starchy vegetables like potatoes and corn

Fiber is also a type of complex carbohydrate and can be found in plant foods. Fiber can help with digestion. The following foods are good sources of fiber:

- Vegetables such as cabbage, spinach, kale
- Fruits like, berries, oranges, apples and peaches with the skin
- Legumes such as chickpeas, black beans, lentils

Certain amounts of fat are also important for your body. During pregnancy, the fats you eat are a source of energy and help with your baby's organs and the placenta. However, be careful not to eat too much saturated fat (such as butter, heavy cream and meats with high content of fat) and trans fat (often found in margarine, microwave popcorn, cookies and pastries made with vegetable shortening) because those can cause problems for your health.

Other nutrients that you need during pregnancy to keep yourself and your baby healthy include:

- Folate or Folic acid. These can help prevent birth defects of the brain and spine in your baby, called neural tube defects. This can be found in enriched and fortified products (like bread, rice, cereals), leafy green vegetables, citrus fruits and beans and peas. Enriched and fortified means the nutrient was added to a food product.
- Calcium. This strengthens bone and teeth for your baby and also helps your body stay healthy during pregnancy. Good sources of calcium are dairy products, broccoli and kale. Fortified cereals or juices may also be a good source.
- Vitamin D. This is also helpful for building your baby's bones and teeth. Good sources include fatty fish like

salmon or fortified milk or orange juice.

- Iron. This helps your body create more blood to help make sure your baby gets enough oxygen. Good sources of iron are meat products and beans. Your body can absorb iron more easily if you also get enough Vitamin C. Vitamin C can be found in orange juice, citrus fruits and strawberries.
- DHA. This is a kind of fat called an omega-3 fatty acid. This is important for the brain and eye development of your baby.
- Iodine. This is a mineral that helps with your baby's brain and nerve growth.

How much should you eat each day during pregnancy?

Most pregnant women need only about 300 extra calories per day during the last 6 months of pregnancy. A glass of skim milk, two small crackers and a tablespoon of peanut butter have approximately 300 calories. The exact amount depends on your weight before pregnancy. If you're underweight before pregnancy, you may need more calories. If you're overweight before, you may need less. Talk to your provider about what's right for you.

Important Reminders During Your Pregnancy

It doesn't matter whether you are a first-timer or well familiar with pregnancy–you need to evaluate your diet for each pregnancy. Everything changes when you become pregnant and each pregnancy can be different from the previous one. You may need to re-educate yourself about what foods are good to eat during pregnancy or what foods to avoid while pregnant.

Professional assistance plays an important role in ensuring you and your child's safety. It would help if you have someone you can call whenever you have questions or concerns regarding your diet or condition; someone to guide you throughout or warn you against bad eating decisions, big or small.

Below are some of the things you need to consider when eating:

- Food sensitivity is common during pregnancy. Apart from pregnancy, you may have underlying medical conditions that would require you to take extra precautions with your diet. In these cases, having a prenatal care specialist is highly recommended.
- Food allergies do not take a break and neither do food cravings. Often, you will feel hungry now that you are eating for two. Increased hunger means an increased risk of developing

food allergies. Your local perinatal dietitian or nutritionist will recommend the best alternatives so you can avoid certain foods that might cause allergic reactions.

- Cooking your meals thoroughly is a good rule of thumb, especially when you are pregnant. Your immune system is affected during pregnancy so the risk for food borne illnesses is higher for you and your unborn child. Proper food preparation is one way of protecting yourself and your baby from health risks.

Chapter 4.

Foods that don't build a healthy conception

Trying to conceive can be a difficult and frustrating process. You're probably doing everything you can to increase your chances, but did you know that there are certain foods you should avoid while trying to conceive? While you may think that what you eat doesn't matter, the truth is that certain foods can actually affect your chances of conceiving.

Diet is an essential part of maintaining and boosting your fertility. A fertility diet is important for everyone trying to conceive but even more so for people who are facing infertility issues such as low sperm count or sperm motility and irregular ovulation due to Polycystic ovary Syndrome (PCOS) and other ovulatory disorders.

Food can help male fertility as well as female fertility but what should you certainly avoid, you ask? Well, in this blog post, we will explore some of the foods you should avoid while trying to conceive, as well as some alternative options that you should be including to maintain your reproductive health and boost your chances to conceive. Read on!

Why is Diet Important for Fertility?

When you're trying to conceive, you're likely to hear a lot of advice about what to eat and what to avoid. Some of it is conflicting, and some of it may even seem contradictory. The truth is, there is no one "right" diet for fertility.

However, eating a healthy diet is important for both men and women who are trying to conceive. There are a few key reasons why a healthy diet is important for fertility.

- Eating a healthy diet helps to ensure that your body is getting the nutrients it needs to function optimally. This includes nutrients like folic acid, which is important for preventing birth defects and reducing the risk of ovulatory infertility.
- Maintaining a healthy weight is important for fertility. Being overweight or underweight can lead to hormonal imbalances that can make it difficult to conceive. A good diet can help with weight gain or weight loss.
- A healthy diet can help reduce stress levels, which can also impact fertility. High levels of stress can interfere with ovulation in women and lower sperm quality and sperm count in men.

- It can help you balance the risk of insulin resistance. In women suffering from PCOS, high blood sugar can lead to diabetes as the action of insulin is restricted. Insulin resistance can lead to a higher risk of diabetes in the long run and can also interfere with menstrual cycles and ovulation.

- What you eat can affect your vaginal pH levels. Having an imbalance in vaginal pH can make it more difficult for sperm to survive and reach the egg. Eating foods that promote vaginal health, like yogurt and cranberries, can help maintain a healthy pH balance.

What Foods to Avoid While Trying to Get Pregnant?

Caffeine

There are many foods and drinks that can affect fertility, and caffeine is one of them. Caffeine can interfere with a woman's ability to conceive by affecting the way her body absorbs and metabolizes nutrients. It can also increase the risk of miscarriage and other pregnancy complications.

Caffeine is found in coffee, tea, energy drinks, chocolate, and some over-the-counter medications. If you're trying to conceive, it's important to limit your caffeine intake or avoid it altogether. Talk to your doctor about how much caffeine is safe for you to consume during pregnancy.

Alcohol

When trying to conceive, it is important to avoid alcohol. Alcohol can reduce fertility in both men and women. It can also increase the risk of miscarriage and birth defects. If you are trying to conceive, it is best to abstain from alcohol entirely.

Alcohol has adverse effects on libido as well as sexual function in men. In women, it throws off the hormone balance in their bodies and can also interfere with normal menstrual cycles making it difficult to get pregnant.

Processed Foods

Processed foods are a big no-no when you're trying to conceive. That's because they're typically high in unhealthy fats, salt, and sugar, and low in the nutrients that are essential for a healthy pregnancy. Processed foods can lead to lower semen quality in men and it is also associated with an increased risk of inflammation in the body. Inflammation is bad news when you're trying to conceive.

So what counts as processed food? Basically, anything that's been through more than one step of processing before it reaches your plate. This includes things like frozen meals, lunch meats, pre-made soups, crackers, and even some so-called "healthy" snacks like granola bars or yogurt drinks.

While you don't have to be perfect when it comes to avoiding processed foods, do your best to limit them as much as possible. Stick with whole, unprocessed foods like fruits, vegetables, lean animal protein, and whole grains. These will give you the nutrients you need for a healthy pregnancy—and help you avoid those extra pounds that can be so tough to lose after the baby arrives. Whole foods ultimately reduce the chance of obesity as well and provide you with a wealth of important elements like omega-3 fatty acids, antioxidants, and essential vitamins like vitamin c . vitamin d, and vitamin b12.

High-mercury Fish

High-mercury fish are one of the foods to avoid while trying to conceive. Mercury is a heavy metal that can damage the nervous system and is especially harmful to developing fetuses. The FDA recommends that women who are pregnant or may become pregnant avoid eating high-mercury fish such as shark, swordfish, king mackerel, and tilefish. Instead, they should eat up to 12 ounces (two average meals) per week of a variety of fish and shellfish that are lower in mercury. These include shrimp, pollock, and salmon.

Unhealthy Fats

There are a few types of fats that can be harmful to your health and should be avoided while trying to conceive. Trans fats, saturated fats, and omega-6 fatty acids can all contribute to inflammation in the body, which can lead to problems with fertility.

Trans fats are found in processed foods like cookies, crackers, and margarine. They can also be found in some fast food. Saturated fats are found in animal products like meat and dairy. They can also be found in coconut oil, palm oil, and other vegetable oils. Omega-6 fatty acids are found in corn oil, soybean oil, and sunflower oil.

Eating a diet high in healthy fats like olive oil, avocados, nuts, and seeds is a good way to make sure you're getting the nutrients you need without exposing yourself to unhealthy fats. It's also a good idea to replace your low-fat dairy with full-fat dairy or whole milk. Low-fat dairy has been found to reduce fertility in men and women while high-fat dairy has been found to help.

High-sugar Drinks and Soda

High-sugar foods and drinks lower fertility in both men and women. It can cause inflammation and also causes the aging of our internal organs including the reproductive system. It has also been linked to lower-quality eggs. Sugary drinks and foods have also been found to affect the success rates of In-vitro fertilization (IVF). By reducing the number of viable eggs and oocytes that can be retrieved, the consumption of sugary drinks can reduce the chances of getting pregnant.

While trying to conceive, it is important to pay attention to the foods you are eating. Some foods can increase the risk of infertility or cause problems during pregnancy. If you are trying to get pregnant, avoid alcohol, caffeine, processed meats, and unpasteurized dairy products. Eating a healthy diet full of fruits, vegetables, and whole grains will help you conceive and have a healthy pregnancy.

Routinely getting tested to understand the nutrient levels in your body, taking necessary supplements, and adjusting your dietary patterns accordingly are the best bet. Along with a good diet, it is also important to focus on your mental and spiritual well-being as well as getting regular exercise and good sleep will also help you boost fertility.

Chapter 5.

Fertility Meal plans

A fertility diet plan is a helpful element of preconception care. Understanding the impact certain foods have on fertility will help you create a plan that will improve your chances of natural conception and a healthy pregnancy.

Why is a fertility diet plan important?

Nutrition is an important part of preconception care. Having a fertility diet plan is great for getting you into healthy habits and preparing your body for pregnancy!

Part of the reason for a fertility diet plan is to help improve your chances of conceiving naturally. Having a generally healthy lifestyle, including a healthy balanced diet Vitamins and minerals will help keep your body's systems incheck – including your reproductive system.

When trying for a baby, it's a good idea to try and reach a healthy BMI. A balanced diet and regular exercise should help you maintain a healthy BMI that's neither too high nor too low. You should aim to have a healthy BMI when trying to conceive. If you have a high BMI, try not to worry too much or be too hard on yourself. It can be difficult to lose weight, and you need to do it with the right support. Being underweight can also impact fertility. Having a low BMI can cause your periods to become more irregular or stop all together.

Inspiration for your diet
For more inspiration to help you get in to a healthy lifestyle, we have lots of blogs on the subject. Check out our advice on exercise for fertility, or if yoga is more your thing, we have an illustrated guide of yoga asanas for fertility.

A woman's diet around the time of conception can also influence the development of her baby. During the first few months of pregnancy the foundations for organ and tissues begin – this is a critical period of development'. During this time the main nutrient supply for the growing fetus comes from the mother's blood, therefore a lack of certain nutrients may impact on the health of the growing baby.

To ensure the best outcome for you and your child it is important to optimize your diet- both before conception and during pregnancy.

How do you create a fertility diet plan?

The foundations of a healthy preconception diet is balance. This is not a crash diet, or solely about you losing weight, This is about you getting the nutrients you need to prepare your body for a healthy pregnancy. However, there are a few foods that can boost your fertility – so you may want to add a few extra portions of those to your plate.

What foods should you eat to increase fertility?
Here are a few key food groups that have nutritional benefits that could help increase both male and female fertility.

Leafy Greens – Dark leafy greens are a great source of calcium, iron and folate. Folate is incredibly important for pregnancy as it helps reduce the risk of certain birth defects.

Try to include a good serving of spinach, kale or swiss chard in your daily diet.

Avocados – Another great source of folate is avocados. It also has Vitamin K, which helps your body absorb nutrients, and potassium which helps regulate blood pressure. Whilst avocados aren't low in fat, they are full of good fats, which our body needs. Try some on a piece of multigrain toast!

Nuts – Nuts are a rich source of protein and walnuts in particular are great for both male and female fertility. They are high in magnesium which for women boost progesterone production and blood flow to the uterus. Walnuts are also thought you improve the shape and vitality of sperm.

Quinoa – Whole grains, like quinoa, are a great source of fiber. They are also packed full of zinc, folate and protein. Plant based proteins are better for you than animal based ones, and can improve your chances of conception. They are thought to help regulate your cycle.

Fish – Most fish, but especially oily fish like salmon, is a wonderful source of omega 3. Omega 3 is important for fetal brain and eye development, so it's a great thing to eat when trying to conceive when or pregnant.

The best fruits for fertility

All fruits are full of nutrients that make them an important part of a fertility diet plan. However, there are a few superfruits that you should definitely try to eat once a day.

Citrus fruits are the best source of vitamin C as well as folate – which is incredibly important for preconception. They are also packed with calcium and potassium. You should try to eat an orange or a grapefruit every day – alongside some other servings of fruit and veg.

Berries are another amazing fruit for anyone trying to conceive. Like citrus fruits, they are full of vitamin D and folate. However, berries like raspberries and blueberries are also loaded with antioxidants and have antiinflammatory properties – which helps both female and male fertility.

Chapter 6.

Supplements

What supplements should I take to increase fertility?
A well-balanced diet will provide you with nearly everything you need for your pregnancy. However, the National Institute of Health and Care Excellence (NICE) recommends that women supplement their diet with two extra vitamins around the time of conception.

Folate – (the natural form of folic acid) is a B-vitamin. It occurs naturally in dark green leafy vegetables, fruits, dairy products and seafood. Low folate status is common in the

UK, and if it occurs during pregnancy it can have a negative impact on babies. They may be born small for their age or have birth defects. The most common defects related to low folate are neural tube defects such as spina bifida.

All women in the UK are advised to take 400ug of folic acid 8 weeks prior to conception. They should then continue taking it up to 12 weeks of pregnancy. This is to ensure there is a good folic acid supply at conception and until the neural tube closes.

Vitamin D – Similarly to folate, vitamin D deficiency is common in the UK. It plays an important role in our bodies, helping with the absorption of dietary calcium and phosphate from our intestines. These three nutrients are needed to help maintain healthy bones, teeth and muscles. They are also key to the development of your baby during pregnancy.

NICE recommends that all women take a daily supplement of 10 ug from conception all the way through their pregnancy. It is also recommended to continue supplementation throughout breastfeeding as well, to ensure there is an adequate supply in breastmilk.

Chapter 7.

stress and mental health

Is There a Connection Between Conception and Your Mental Health?

Taking care of your mental and emotional health is just as important as your physical health when you're trying to get pregnant.

When you decide to try to get pregnant, it's a great time to start preparing your body to conceive and carry a healthy baby. But taking care of yourself isn't all about physical health. For some, the journey of getting pregnant can take time (and can potentially feel stressful and frustrating), so focusing on your mental and emotional health is super important too!

Can Mental Health Conditions Affect My Chances of Getting Pregnant?

They can. But at the same time...they might not. As with so many things in regard to fertility and conception, the truth is that it's different for every woman. However, it's true that there are a lot of different factors that can affect the regularity of your periods and menstrual cycle (and therefore getting pregnant) including your mental health.

Studies show that certain mental health disorders such as anxiety disorder, clinical depression, bipolar disorder and eating disorders are linked to irregular or shortened periods. Another culprit of irregular periods? Stress. Research shows that high levels of long-term (or chronic) stress can also contribute to irregular periods, as it affects the part of your brain that controls reproduction.

Short or irregular periods can make it difficult to track your cycle and pinpoint when your body ovulates, which can therefore make it harder for you and your partner to know when to try to conceive.

Should I Continue Taking Medication for My Mental Health Condition While Trying to Get Pregnant?

This is an important conversation you'll need to have with your provider. The truth of the matter is that every person's situation is different. While some medicines (such as certain antidepressants) could make it difficult for you to get pregnant, the benefits of taking them for your mental health may outweigh the risks of stopping your medicine. Whatever path you and your provider decide to take, do not stop taking medication without your provider's approval. They will advise you how to stop your medication in the healthiest way, or even switch you to a medication that is safer for pregnant mamas and their growing babies.

When you decide to try to get pregnant, one of the first things you should do is to schedule a pre-pregnancy checkup with your provider. During this appointment, you and your provider will discuss your medical history and make a plan on how to best manage your mental health—all while encouraging conception and a healthy pregnancy.

If you're trying to get pregnant and feeling stressed or worried about your chances of conceiving, the truth is that this has the potential to negatively impact your mental health. It's important to keep in touch with your provider, therapist and your partner (or any support person) about your feelings throughout the process. Taking good care of your mental health is one of the most important things you can do as you head into motherhood (and beyond).

lost the baby around the second trimester.

"It's so stressful when you don't know why you're having trouble," says Chaimovitz, now 42. "I wanted a baby so badly I would have hung upside down or drunk gallons of green juice if I thought it helped."

So Chaimovitz eagerly signed up for the mindfulness program led by Alice Domar, PhD, executive director of the Domar Center for Mind/Body Health. The 10-week sessions included yoga, meditation, and learning behavioral techniques like overcoming negative thoughts. Several months after finishing the program, Chaimovitz got pregnant again. Her daughter, Romi, was born in 2018.

"When you're trying to get pregnant and someone tells you to just relax, you get annoyed," Chaimovitz says. "But in my case,

I really do think it helped. I stopped feeling like my body was the enemy."

It's not easy to tease out all the reasons why some couples seem to conceive easily and quickly while others have much more trouble. But research suggests that stress may be one factor that can affect the concept of math.

The Science Behind Stress and Fertility

Several recent studies have found links between the women's levels of day-to-day stress and lowered chances of pregnancy. For example, women whose saliva had high levels of alpha-amylase, an enzyme that marks stress, took 29% longer to get pregnant compared to those who had less.

"Your body is smart, it knows that (periods of stress) aren't good times to have a baby," says Domar, a longtime infertility researcher who also is director of mind/body services at Boston IVF.

At the same time, stressed women probably also have sex less often, Domar says. And they may be more likely to smoke or drink too much alcohol or caffeine -- behaviors that can hardly improve their odds.

Domar faced skepticism when she published a small study in 1990 showing that lowering stress with group therapy, individual cognitive behavior therapy, and relaxation techniques like guided imagery helped some infertile women get pregnant.

"The medical community said I was stupid to believe that the mind had any control over the ovaries," Domar recalls.

Domar followed that with a much bigger study a decade later to report that among women who had trouble conceiving, those who received cognitive behavioral therapy were almost twice as likely to end up pregnant as those who didn't.

Today, researchers widely accept that stress and fertility are connected.

"We know now that stress hormones such as cortisol disrupt signaling between the brain and the ovaries, which can trip up ovulation," says Sarah Berga, MD, an infertility specialist and vice chair of women's health at Wake Forest Medical Center in Winston-Salem, N.C.

Tackling Stress

Everyone gets stressed once in a while. So if you're frazzled for a few weeks at work or feel anxious about a big move, it likely won't hurt your baby-making abilities. But if your stress goes on for a long time or if you're dealing with a major upheaval like unemployment or a death in the family, then your ovulation might get thrown out of whack, Berga says.

About 1 in 10 women of childbearing age have trouble conceiving or finishing the pregnancy, according to the CDC. Usually, there is a physical reason, such as blocked fallopian tubes.

But as months go by without conception, stress may kick in.

"Women struggling with infertility have the same levels of anxiety and depression as women diagnosed with cancer or HIV," Domar says. As a result, a vicious cycle starts.

Domar's mind/body program aims to curb that stress through several approaches. First is talk therapy to help reframe your feelings. You learn to challenge automatic negative thoughts like, "I'll never get pregnant," or blaming yourself.

Domar's clients also practice a type of yoga called hatha yoga, which pairs yoga postures with deep breathing exercises. She says it's a way for women to nurture themselves.

 "A lot of my patients are angry at their bodies, so they stop taking care of it," Domar says. "This is a way for them to feel connected to themselves again."

Domar says it's also important for the women and their partners to talk and to listen to each other about their shared struggles. That, along with plugging into support groups, can help ease the mental and emotional toll from infertility.

Chapter 8.

Health and lifestyle that impair infertility

Lifestyle Factors That Can Cause Infertility

For the estimated 10-18% of couples affected by infertility, finding the root cause of the problem can be a difficult and lengthy process. That's because, taken on the whole, fertility problems are just as likely to be caused by female factors as male factors — or a combination of both.

Many of the women and couples who come to see us here at Rodeo Drive Women's

Health Center in Beverly Hills, California, are surprised to learn that their problem isn't the result of an underlying medical condition like low sperm count or polycystic ovary syndrome (PCOS).

In many cases, infertility is the result of lifestyle factors that compromise reproductive health and make pregnancy far less likely.

Fortunately, most of these factors are controllable, meaning they can be altered or reversed simply by making better choices and improving certain daily habits. Read on to learn more about how your lifestyle affects your fertility, and what you can do about it.

Body weight
More than six million women in the United States — or roughly one in 10 women of reproductive age — experience difficulty becoming pregnant or staying pregnant. For

many of these women, infertility is a direct result of being overweight, obese, or significantly underweight.

Being overweight or underweight can make it more difficult to become pregnant because both conditions influence your estrogen levels and disrupt normal ovulation, which is the monthly release of an egg from one of your ovaries.

Regular ovulation requires normal estrogen levels, but being overweight can lead to higher concentrations of circulating estrogen, which acts much like birth control to prevent ovulation. Being underweight, on the other hand, can make it difficult for your body to maintain adequate estrogen levels to support monthly ovulation.

For women on both ends of the spectrum, taking steps toward a healthier weight is often enough to restore normal ovulation and make pregnancy possible.

Nutrition

Although there's limited research on exactly how a woman's nutritional status affects her chances of conceiving, there's plenty of evidence to indicate that eating a nutritious diet supports optimal body functioning and general well-being.

Still, there's no specific "fertility diet" that you should adapt when you're trying to conceive. Instead, remember that your body performs best when it's fueled by the right blend of nutrients, and your reproductive system is no different.

That means choosing whole foods like vegetables, fruits, whole grains, proteins, and healthy fats, while limiting or eliminating refined grain products and foods that are rich in added sugars, preservatives, or unhealthy fats.

It's important to note, however, that untreated celiac disease (gluten intolerance) has been shown to interfere with female fertility.

Physical activity

Exercise is an essential part of maintaining a strong, healthy body, but when you're trying to get pregnant, it's a good idea to avoid excessive physical activity. That's because strenuous exercise can interfere with normal ovulation and reduce your levels of progesterone, a reproductive hormone that's essential for pregnancy.

In fact, researchers have found a strong correlation between increased frequency, intensity, and duration of exercise and decreased fertility in women.

Whether you're trying to lose weight or you've been an athlete all your life, stick with moderate exercise when you're trying to conceive. Women who want to maintain more intense training programs are generally advised to limit vigorous exercise to no more than five hours each week.

Smoking

If you're a smoker and you've been struggling to conceive, you now have one more reason to quit.

Tobacco negatively affects female fertility in a myriad of ways. It can prematurely age your ovaries, deplete your eggs, damage your cervix and fallopian tubes, and increase your risk of having an ectopic pregnancy or miscarriage.

If all of that weren't enough, smoking is also incredibly harmful to a growing fetus and your overall health. Kicking the habit for good can help you overcome fertility problems, protect your pregnancy, and have a healthy baby.

Alcohol consumption

Health experts have long known that drinking any amount of alcohol during pregnancy can be dangerous to an unborn child. More recently, they've also discovered that drinking alcohol can also significantly reduce a woman's fertility.

Although researchers aren't clear on exactly how alcohol undermines conception, evidence suggests it may interfere with normal ovulation on multiple levels.

Because no one knows how much or how little alcohol it takes to interfere with reproductive function, women who are trying to conceive are generally encouraged to avoid alcohol completely.

Other factors

Being overweight, eating an unhealthy diet, working out too hard, smoking cigarettes, and drinking alcohol aren't the only lifestyle factors that can influence your ability to become pregnant.

You may have a harder time getting pregnant if you have anxiety, suffer from depression, or live with some other form of chronic psychological stress. If you feel stressed out more often than not, finding ways to relax or seeking support can make a significant difference.

Your fertility can also be impacted by regular exposure to toxic chemicals. Lead in your drinking water can alter hormone levels and reduce fertility, for example, while many of the chemicals used in pesticides can disrupt normal hormonal activity and interfere with reproductive health.

Fertility experts even recommend limiting the amount of caffeine you consume when trying to conceive, although research hasn't yet shown a clear link between too much caffeine and infertility. Just as with alcohol, however, it's better to be safe than sorry when you're doing everything you can to get pregnant.

Chapter 9.

preconception planning

Starting a family can be one of the most rewarding life experiences. But the journey towards becoming a parent can sometimes feel like navigating uncharted waters. Understanding your body, knowing how to prepare for pregnancy, and learning how to boost your fertility are all essential steps on the path to motherhood.

Every journey is unique. Some people conceive almost immediately, while others may take longer. It's important to remember that there's no 'right' timeline — what matters most is taking steps to optimize your health and well-being to enhance your fertility.

We're here to help guide you through this important life event, providing trusted health advice and products to support you along the way.

General Health Considerations for Prospective Parents

Before you even begin trying for a baby, it's important to prepare your body for this life-changing event. Think of it as setting the stage for the miracle of life to take place. Here's where lifestyle choices play a big role.

Balanced Diet: A diet rich in fruits, vegetables, whole grains, and lean protein provides a balanced mix of essential nutrients. Avoid excessive intake of processed foods and limit caffeine and alcohol.

Exercise Regularly: Physical activity is beneficial not just for your general health but also for reproductive health. Regular exercise can help maintain a healthy weight, which is important for fertility.

Manage Stress: Chronic stress can impact fertility. It's crucial to find stress management techniques that work for you, such as yoga, meditation, or even simple breathing exercises.

Quit Smoking: Smoking affects fertility in both men and women. If you're a smoker, quitting is one of the best things you can do when trying to conceive.

Making these changes can help prepare your body for pregnancy and increase your chances of conceiving. Of course, achieving optimal health doesn't happen overnight, so patience is key.

Timing Matters: Understanding Ovulation and Your Fertility Window

When it comes to making your dreams of motherhood come true, timing is everything. The fertility window, or the optimal time for conception, usually spans a few days in each menstrual cycle. This is typically around ovulation, when an egg is released from the ovaries.

Understanding your own menstrual cycle is essential in predicting this fertility window. A regular menstrual cycle lasts 28 days, but it can range from 21 to 35 days in different women. Ovulation generally happens around the midpoint of the cycle. Observing signs of ovulation, like increased cervical mucus and mild pelvic pain, can also provide clues.

However, these natural signs can sometimes be hard to interpret. That's where ovulation test kits and fertility monitors come in handy. These tools can help pinpoint the timing of ovulation more accurately by detecting hormonal changes in urine or saliva. Used correctly, they can take the guesswork out of your conception journey, improving your chances of successful conception.

Every woman's cycle is unique, and it might take a bit of time to understand your own patterns. Be patient with yourself, and seek professional help if you're having trouble figuring things out.

Predicte Ovulation Strip is designed to help you identify your most fertile days each month.

Preconception Nutrition: Key Supplements for Women Trying to Conceive

When trying to conceive, not only is a balanced diet important, but so is the addition of specific vitamins and minerals. These supplements can help prepare your body for pregnancy and promote the healthy development of your baby.

Folic Acid: Folic acid is a B vitamin that is crucial for the healthy development of the baby's neural tube. It's recommended to start taking a supplement with 400 mcg of folic acid at least one month before you start trying to conceive.

L-Arginine: L-arginine is an amino acid that may enhance fertility by improving blood flow to the reproductive organs. Some studies suggest it can improve ovarian response, endometrial receptivity, and potentially ovarian reserve, in women trying to conceive.

Vitamin D: Some research has linked sufficient levels of Vitamin D to better outcomes in fertility treatments. Adequate levels of Vitamin D can help improve your chances of conceiving and having a healthy pregnancy.

OvaCare Tablets offer balanced micronutrients and vitamins to support fertility and conception. They contain strong folic acid elements and other compounds like Inositol and L-Arginine to improve ovarian function and increase pregnancy rates.

Conception for Her, the prenatal supplement that supports fertility when you're trying to conceive. Formulated with clinically validated ingredients like Myo-Inositol, Chaste Tree Berry, KSM-66® Ashwagandha Extract, and more.

It's important to consult with a healthcare professional before you start any supplement regimen. They can provide personalized advice based on your individual health needs. GoMed has a team of professional pharmacists available via chat to answer any questions and help guide you in your journey to motherhood.

Addressing Potential Fertility Issues: The Harder Conversations

Navigating the path to parenthood can sometimes bring unexpected challenges, and understanding these potential obstacles is crucial for optimal preconception care. Both men and women can face fertility issues, and it's important to approach these potential issues with compassion, knowledge, and the right medical support.

Ovulation Disorders: More Common Than You Think

Ovulation disorders, including Polycystic Ovary Syndrome (PCOS), are a common cause of infertility in women. These disorders can disrupt or eliminate ovulation, which is the release of an egg. Symptoms may include irregular periods or no periods at all, and lifestyle changes, medications, or even assisted reproductive technology can help address these issues.

Exeline Fertilady, helps restore ovulation and aids conception in women with polycystic ovarian syndrome women who have irregular or no ovulation.

Low Sperm Motility in Men

In about a third of cases, infertility is related to the male partner. One of the key parameters of male fertility is sperm mobility or motility - the sperm's ability to move. If mobility is compromised, the sperm may not be able to reach the egg to fertilize it. A variety of factors, including health, lifestyle, and genetic issues, can influence sperm motility.

Addyzoa Capsules are specifically formulated to enhance sperm health and semen density, playing a key role in improving fertility outcomes.

Structural Issues: Tubes and Tissues Matter

In some cases, structural problems can cause or contribute to infertility. In women, these may involve the fallopian tubes or uterus. For men, it could be a blockage in the different ducts that carry sperm. In many of these cases, surgery can correct the problem.

Age-Related Infertility

Age is a major factor affecting fertility, particularly for women. As a woman ages, the number and quality of her eggs decline, which can make conception more difficult. This decline speeds up after the age of 35. For men, sperm quality can decline with age, although the effect on fertility is less direct.

If you think these factors are affecting your chances of having a baby, it is crucial to seek professional medical advice. At GoMed, our licensed healthcare professionals are ready to assist you in your journey.

The Role of Professional Guidance: When to Seek Help

For many, trying to conceive is a journey that can be filled with uncertainty and questions. It's essential to know that you're not alone and professional help is available. If you've been trying to conceive for over a year without success, or for six months if you're over 35, it's typically recommended to consult a healthcare provider. This can help identify potential underlying issues and suggest solutions tailored to your specific situation. For men, it's also crucial to be part of this process, as male fertility issues contribute to around half of all fertility issues.

At GoMed, we're committed to providing accessible, reliable healthcare solutions. Our platform offers a free chat feature that connects you with highly qualified pharmacists to answer your questions, as well as a telemedicine service for consultations with licensed doctors. Whether you're just starting your journey or are further along, we're here to provide the support you need.

Remember, every journey is unique, and there's no one-size-fits-all solution when it comes to fertility. It's about finding what works for you and your partner, and we're here to help you navigate that process.

Supportive Products and Services: Enhancing Your Fertility Journey

Your path to parenthood might be smooth, or it might require a bit of extra assistance. Alongside lifestyle changes and professional advice, certain products and services can enhance your fertility journey.

GoMed offers a wide range of over-the-counter supplements known for supporting fertility, such as folic acid and l-arginine, as well as prenatal vitamins crucial for early pregnancy. Remember, while supplements can play a supportive role, they should be used in conjunction with a healthy lifestyle, and it's always best to consult a healthcare provider before starting any new regimen.

In addition to supplements, our platform also carries a variety of fertility aids like ovulation test kits and fertility monitors, which can help you better understand your cycle and pinpoint your most fertile days.

Chapter 10.

Improving Egg and sperm quality

How to boost egg & sperm quality?

Sperm and egg quality are one of the most important factors when it comes to fertility and getting pregnant. There are plenty of things men can do to improve their sperm count and health. Women, on the other hand, can't do anything about the number of eggs they have left in the ovaries. However, there are a number of proactive steps they can take to improve the quality of their eggs, and by doing so, to make it easier to conceive naturally.

What exactly is sperm and egg quality?

Egg quality refers to the ability of the egg to produce a healthy pregnancy and baby. A normal, healthy egg has 23 chromosomes and when combined with sperm (which also has 23 chromosomes), it creates an embryo (fertilized egg) containing 46 chromosomes in total.

Sperm quality is defined as the ability of sperm to accomplish fertilization. Whether sperm will fertilize a mature egg or not depends on the following three main factors:

number of sperm (sperm count)
shape of sperm (morphology)
movement of sperm (motility)

What can cause low sperm quality?

Various health issues can contribute to low-quality sperm, including:

Hypothalamic dysfunction
Pituitary gland disorders
Testicular disorders
Sperm transportation problems
Age (especially after age 50)
Lifestyle and environmental factors

Factors that negatively affect egg quality

Egg cells are very fragile and can be easily affected by both internal and external factors, such as:

Age (especially after age 35)
Genetics (e.g. low egg count at birth, early menopause)
Toxic environmental exposures
Prolonged stress
Unhealthy lifestyle habits
Medical conditions (e.g. cancer)
Some medical procedures (e.g. ovarian surgery, cancer treatment)
Weight outside the normal BMI

Things to do to improve your egg quality

While there may be things outside of your control, start by understanding and targeting the factors that negatively affect your egg quality.

Lifestyle
Your lifestyle can have a positive or negative impact on your fertility, so make sure you make better choices, like:

Eating healthily
Avoiding cigarettes and alcohol
Achieving/maintaining a normal BMI
Consider complementary therapies
Acupuncture has been shown to improve blood flow, which in return can improve the flow of oxygen and nutrients to the ovaries (and egg cells). Other benefits of acupuncture include reducing stress, relieving pain and improving mood.

Egg quality improving foods

Eating as if you're already pregnant can actually help prepare your body for pregnancy. If you're trying to conceive, consider including the following foods on your menu:

Avocados
Beans and lentils
Nuts and dry fruits
Sesame seeds
Berries
Green leafy vegetables
Ginger
Supplements for egg health

Supplements that can improve the quality of your eggs include:

Folic acid
Zinc
Selenium
CoQ10
DHEA
Vitamin C, B, E and D

Fish oil and omega-3 fatty acids

Ways to improve sperm quality
There are also a number of ways you can improve your chances of becoming a dad.

Lifestyle
Following a pro-fertility lifestyle will help you avoid nutrient deficiencies or low testosterone levels, which may contribute to infertility. These include:

Exercising regularly
Sleeping 7-8 hours each night
Limiting stress
Avoiding saunas and hot tubs
Sperm-boosting foods

These foods will give your sperm a boost and will improve your chances of conceiving:

Avocado
Asparagus

Broccoli
Green leafy vegetables
Lentils and beans
Salmon, cod, haddock
Meat
Seafood
Olive oil
Walnuts
Citrus fruits
Dark chocolate

Supplements to increase sperm count
Supplements that have been shown to positively affect sperm count include:

D-aspartic acid (D-AA)
Coenzyme Q10
Vitamin E, C and D
Calcium
Zinc
Multi-antioxidant supplement
N-acetyl-cysteine
Selenium
What if I have low-quality eggs or sperm?

Poor egg/sperm quality does not necessarily mean you cannot get pregnant. There are couples who despite having low-quality eggs or zero sperm count still managed to successfully get pregnant and give birth to a healthy child. However, if you're having difficulty getting pregnant, it is important to consult a fertility expert. They will order tests to get an accurate picture of your medical situation and will provide guidance so you make informed family decisions.

Treatment options for low sperm and egg quality

Based on the test results and your medical history, our doctor may recommend one of the following treatment options for infertility:

Treatments for women

IVF

During an in vitro fertilization (IVF) cycle, women with poor quality eggs will be administered hormonal injections followed by an egg retrieval procedure. At this point, patients may decide to fertilize or freeze their eggs.

Egg donor IVF
Egg donor IVF is another treatment option for women with low-quality eggs. High-quality donor eggs are fertilised by the male partner's (or donor) sperm and are either implanted or stored for future use.

Additional treatment options may include hormonal therapy or surgery.

Treatments for men
IVF with ICSI
With IVF, eggs are fertilized in a special laboratory and are then transferred to the patient's uterus to establish a pregnancy. Intracytoplasmic sperm injection (ICSI) is a sophisticated technique that successfully overcomes low sperm count and sperm quality issues. Using ICSI, individual sperm

cells are injected into each mature egg to achieve fertilization.

Sperm donor IVF
Men facing severe male-factor infertility (e.g. azoospermia) are often recommended IVF with donor sperm. The eggs are fertilized with sperm from the chosen donor through ICSI. The best embryo is then transferred to the female partner's uterus or is frozen for future treatment cycles.

Other approaches may include hormonal therapy or surgery.

Start your journey to parenthood today!
If getting pregnant is your top priority, it is important that you and your partner look after your reproductive health, which starts from your egg and sperm. Before changing your diet or lifestyle, talk to a doctor, nutritionist or fertility specialist.

If after twelve months of trying (or six months, if you are over 35) you're still unable to conceive, seek help from a fertility specialist. Based on the results of your infertility evaluation, our EuroCARE IVF specialist will recommend the best treatment for you (and your partner), so that you can achieve your dream of parenthood.

www.ingramcontent.com/pod-product-compliance
Lightning Source LLC
Chambersburg PA
CBHW071224260726
48653CB00042B/2305